What You Need to Know about Healthy Foods

Tips on Getting the Full Benefits from Healthy Foods

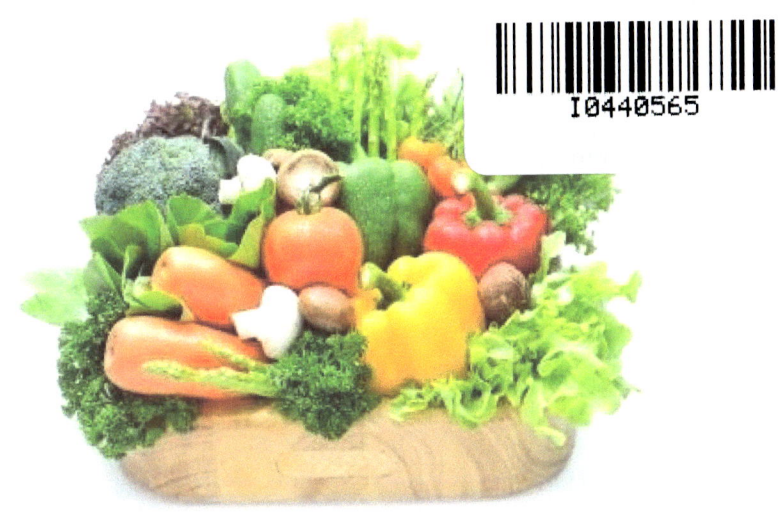

Health Learning Series

Dueep Jyot Singh

Mendon Cottage Books

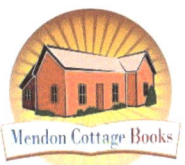

JD-Biz Publishing

Check out some of the other Health Learning Series books at Amazon.com

Health Learning Series on Amazon

Download Free Books!

http://MendonCottageBooks.com

Table of Contents

Introduction

Why were our ancestors so healthy? How did Methuselah live 900 years? How did our ancestors manage spans of longevity, when they were not influenced by wars and disease? Well, the answer is very clear. They were extremely careful about their diet. The ancient wise men advocated a diet of fruit and vegetables, fresh from the trees, and less of high-protein, in the shape of animals, fish and game.

However, as time went by, man began changing his dietary habits. He started domesticating animals, which included poultry, cattle and other animals from where he could get protein supplements in the shape of meat. And so as time went by, he began concentrating more on meat dishes to add variety to his food, rather than plant products.

So as centuries went by, this change in diet slowly and steadily began to have an adverse effect on his health. He started eating less vegetables and fruit, and started concentrating more on protein from animal products. And so his system and physiology began to change accordingly. Nature tried its best to incorporate this change in diet into his natural system. If man had it his way, he would subsist only on meat with less of fruit and vegetables.

However, the wise men were still intelligent enough to make man understand that he needed a natural balance of healthy carbohydrates, proteins, minerals, and other essential nutrients, which could not be obtained by eating just a one-sided diet concentrating on just one particular food group.

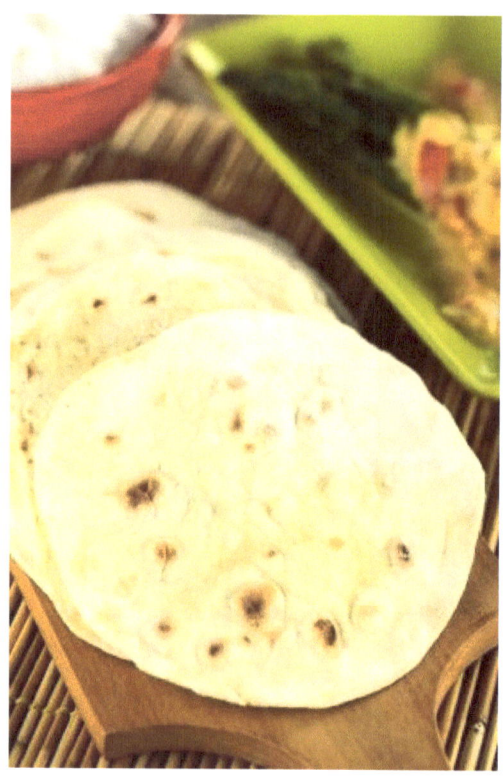

Ordinary bread was the easiest way in which man got his quota of cereals every day. This whole wheat or grain bread was cooked on a grill and eaten with vegetables and meat dishes.

And so they began to tell people more about how necessary it was to eat healthy, beneficial healthy giving foods. These needed to be eaten every day, so that the body could function normally and properly to keep it in proper healthy running condition.

Scarcity of these healthy giving foods would give rise to ailments which would weaken the body. Luckily, man was practical enough to understand the wisdom of such knowledge. And that is why down the millenniums we are still eating fruit and vegetables, herbs and spices.

You may say that you know how to choose, cook and preserve a number of foods given in this book. But there are still some helpful tips, which are going to come in useful, when preparing healthy meals for your family. Naturally the tips are time tested!

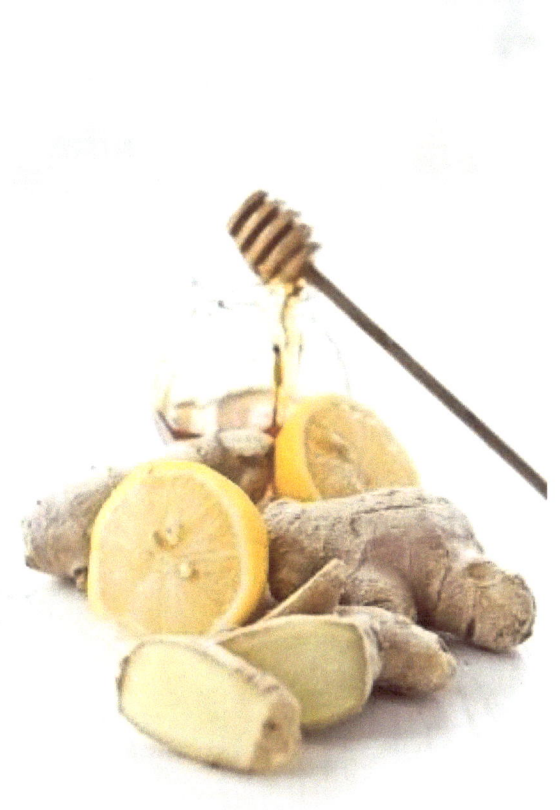

Sugar is not a substitute for honey.

So here are some healthy giving and healing foods, which you need to have in your daily diet, to keep you bright eyed and bushy tailed. And naturally, nuts come in this category.

Some of these foods are vegetarian and some of them are non-vegetarian. So it depends upon your eating habits, which of them you incorporate in your daily diet. But remember that no food can be compensated with another food.

Every single food item in the world has its own unique properties. So if you think that eating lots of honey instead of beetroot sugar is going to keep you healthy, no, that cannot be done, and vice versa. That is, of course, if you are trying to cure yourself of an ailment, where the doctor recommended honey and you're trying to make do with Demerara or molasses. Because after all, all of them are sweet, aren't they.

This sort of thinking is specious and erroneous.

So we start with vegetarian foods –

Organically Grown Fresh Green Vegetables

Fresh green vegetables are the best source of micronutrients for you. As children, we did not mind walking into the kitchen and chomping on any green vegetables, which had been harvested fresh from the garden and was placed there on the slab for cooking.

But then, since childhood, we had learned that fresh fruit and vegetables were fun to crunch. We were very surprised when we found out that there were fussy eaters who hated the thought of greens and yellows and reds, and anything which came in vegetable form.

Spinach was one of the pet abominations of some of my classmates. So when I told them, "I think nobody knows how to cook spinach in your house, the way our grandmother cooks them, it's just wonderful" they decided that must be so. That was because their mothers could not care less about making the dish tasty, because they were in such a hurry doing other things throughout the day.

This is one of the main reasons why so many people do not learn to appreciate green vegetables during childhood. That is because kale, broccoli, mustard greens, and other fresh leafy green vegetables are not added to the vegetable list, when mama goes shopping. And if she has an organic garden, she is not going to plant them, because it is such a problem cooking them. You have to harvest the leaves, remove them from the stalks, wash them, chop them, cook them, and then spice and season them.

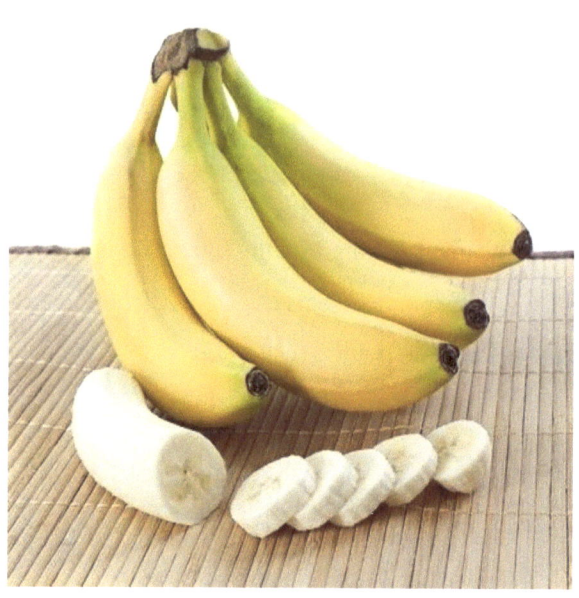

Fast to eat, healthy, and delicious!

Who wants to take all this trouble? Feed your kids ready-made meals and TV dinners instead.

Even if you hate cooking, you may want to try homemade soups with green leafy vegetables. Add some tomatoes, chives, salt, your preferred spices and seasonings, lemon juice, a swirl of cream and chopped parsley for garnish and eat with garlic bread. You may find yourself becoming a green leafy vegetable addict.

Once a week, I can't resist junk food. A whole week of healthy eating and I need to break out with something really chunky and junky. So my version of a hamburger with lots of ketchup and mustard is always one layer of meat products – ham, salami or a grilled hamburger –, one layer of cheese, one layer of tomato-I lightly grill the slices on a griddle so that I do not have a soggy burger –, 3-4 green leaves of any available salad, – lettuce or cabbage- a dab of butter, and homemade mayonnaise with lots of mustard.

Definitely hits the right spots, especially when I taste the contrast of cheese with ham and greens. Then I sprinkled my favorite spices like Oregano, pepper, garlic – salt, chili powder, Sage, Rosemary, basil and thyme on the giant over piled hamburger. Multiplied by 3 – 4, if I'm really hungry. And I'm all set for the day.

No wonder the Danish smorgasbords are such an eclectic mixture of greens, cheeses, and meats. And no wonder they have a weight problem, because they are always confronted with such delicious combinations of flavor, taste, and textures.

I think it is the greens, which makes this crunchy, munchy, dish so delicious, because otherwise, I would not eat greens so often.

So increase the quantity of green leafy vegetables in your meals, and enjoy the difference.

Choosing Vegetables

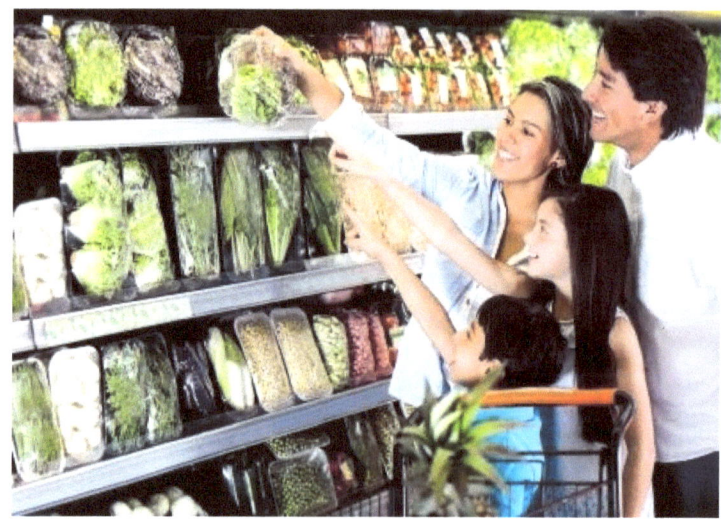

Choose a variety of vegetables because they all differ in appearance, cost, taste and food values.

Choose green and yellow vegetables frequently and those that can be served raw.

Frozen vegetables should be chosen only as a last resort, and depending to season, cost and time available for preparation.

Choose the fresh vegetables for brightness of color, blemish free appearance, no soft spots, and discoloration. Choose them in that amount and quantity that can be stored properly and he used while the quality of the vegetable is still high and fresh.

How to Store Vegetables

Store the fresh vegetables for as short a time as possible in a cool moist, dark place. An exception is onions, which keep better in dry storage

Wash the salad vegetables, trim, if necessary, drain and store in a vegetables crisper or in plastic bags in the refrigerator.

I normally leave fresh corn in the husks and peas in the pod. I store them in the refrigerator until they are ready to use.

Remove the tops off beets and carrots, wash, trim, and store in a cool place. You can save the fresh beetroot tops and cook them like spinach.

Frozen vegetables should be put in the freezer as quickly as possible after purchase. You can cook them without pre-thawing. An exception is corn on the cob, which has to be defrosted before cooking.

Right tips For Boiling Vegetables

Put your vegetables in boiling water. Use just a little water. Simmer until the vegetables are tender crisp. Overcooking and wasting heat by rapid boiling is going to make your vegetables soggy and overcooked. Using a lot of water is wasteful. Use the cooking liquid for gravies. Throwing cooking liquid down the drain means that you are wasting valuable mineral resources.

I found this vegetable cooking chart very helpful and useful. This site also has some good tips on microwaving and blanching vegetables.

http://recipes.howstuffworks.com/tools-and-techniques/how-to-cook-vegetables24.htm

Cook only until the vegetables are tender. Overcooking is going to reduce the color and flavor and is often responsible for turning people against vegetables. Whole potatoes and beets require a little more water. Leafy green vegetables will cook over moderate heat in the water, which clings to the washed leaves. That is how I cook spinach. Absolutely no water.

The color of green vegetables can be preserved better, if the pan is uncovered for 2 or 3 minutes at the beginning. I normally put some salt in peas to keep the color.

Pressure Cooking

This is the cooking method which is not often found in many parts of the world. I have found an easy way to cook vegetables in a pressure cooker by watching the clock very carefully.

Just put diced carrots, cauliflower, and peas with half a teaspoonful of salt in 6 tablespoons water. Now allow the pressure to build up for exactly 3 minutes on low heat. Switch off, but do not lift off the lid. The rest of the cooking is going to be done through steam cooking, and before you utilize the vegetables.

This also does not give me squashy squidgy peas.

Cook until they are just tender. Drain. Use the liquid for gravy or in a sauce. Season to taste, add butter if desired, and serve at once.

Baking and grilling vegetables

Bake the vegetables, whole or even grated in a moderate oven at 350°F. Potatoes may be baked in a hot oven at 425°F. Or they may be parboiled and placed in a pan with a roast at 325°F.

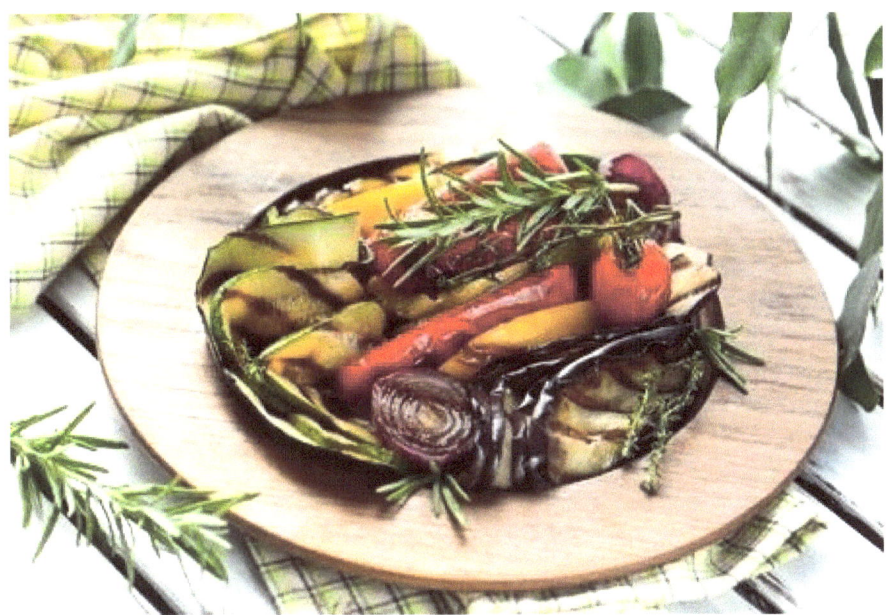

You can convert Fahrenheit into Celsius on this URL.

http://www.onlineconversion.com/temperature.htm.

The web owner also has a downloadable converter.

Slice, dice or greater vegetables like carrots and parsnips for baking in a covered casserole with a little bit of water or butter and seasonings to taste. Bake until they are just tender.

Steaming vegetables

This method takes longer than boiling, or pressure cooking, but retains appearance and flavor. Place the prepared vegetables in a perforated section of a steamer, over boiling water, cover and cook until just tender. Season and serve at once. This is a good method for cooking the vegetables for a stew. The meat is going to simmer in the lower section of steamer and the prepared vegetables cook in the perforated section.

Steaming Fish Episode

My father, who enjoys healthy cooking and does not have many teeth, discovered steaming for cooking fish just a couple of weeks ago! These 80 + years, he had spent eating fish, fried, baked, barbecued, in curries or roasted, but now he is thrilled with steamed fish, which he can eat without dentures.

He found that boiling fish or meat in order to soften it spoiled its taste and also made it hard. That was unless he made a stew, when the meat would be cooked for about 4 to 5 hours until it fell away into a mushy delicious fragrant stew

So one day he put the fish on a perforated rack with extremely small holes.

He borrowed the rack from the oven, where it had been given as an accessory for grilling, when that Baby Belling was bought in England, more than 60 years ago.

I do not know if you can find such a rack easily nowadays, in the market, but he bent it to make it fit in the pressure cooker. So now he has a rack with holes the size of a fine grater.

Anyway, here were the pieces of fish placed on that perforated rack. The water below was just enough to prevent the pressure cooker from drying out. 2 ½ inches is adequate, as long as it does not touch the fish.

Salt the water, add some herbs and spices for seasoning, pieces of garlic, – hey, you are going to be getting spicy soup – water, as a result of this steaming – and put the pressure pan lid on. This will now be steamed on slow heat to give you deliciously soft steamed fish.

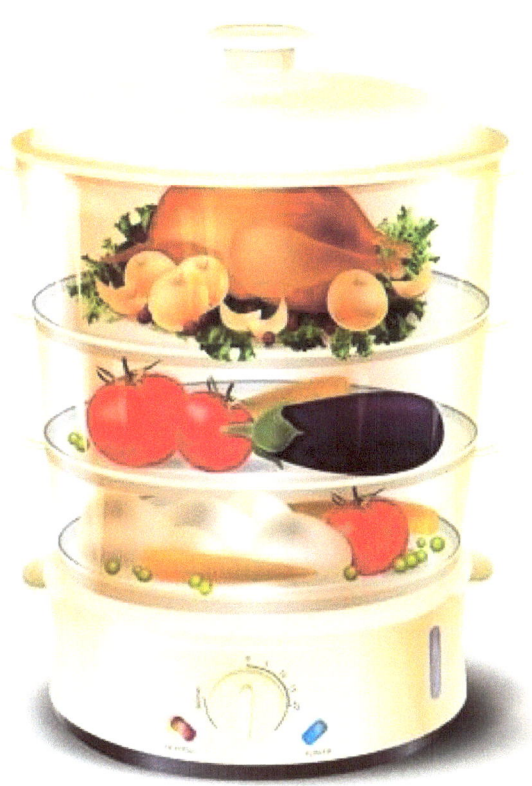

And then he went off to watch National Geographic Channel for the next 30 minutes. After that, he got up, switched off the heat and allowed the fish to steam cook in the condensed cooling steam for another 10 minutes or so.

Delicious, healthy steamed fish was ready for him, when he decided it was time for lunch.

This creamy delicious fish just crumbled away at his touch and went down as smooth as silk.

Some days ago, he also tried steaming pieces of tough pork meat, which he could not chew otherwise, when it was cooked fried. When boiled, it got all tough and leathery. No fun. Also, red meat pork chops had to be marinated to soften them for about 48 hours before he barbecued them. Even so, they were so tough to chew.

Steaming softened that meat wonderfully well. [No, he does not steam pork chops. That would be such a sad waste!]

So now, one has another extremely helpful and useful cooking method, with which one can eat healthy foods, even when one is sans teeth.

Cooking Frozen Vegetables

Add the frozen vegetables except corn on the cob to a small amount of boiling water over high heat. Breakup the block with a fork as it begins to thaw. When the water returns to the boil, reduce heat and boil gently until just tender. Frozen vegetables require less cooking than fresh ones – from ½ to 2/3 of the time.

Suitable frozen vegetables may be sealed in aluminum foil or placed in a tightly covered casserole with seasonings and butter and baked in a moderate over until just tender.

You can also cook them on an outdoor grill, if they are foil– wrapped.

Heating canned vegetables

Canned vegetables are already cooked and only need to be thoroughly heated for serving. You can do that in your microwave. Or you can cook them by pouring the liquid from the can into the saucepan and heat to boiling. Nowadays, there are many companies which allow you to heat food in the can itself. But of course you are not going to put this metal can into the microwave.

You can add vegetables and leave over moderate heat until it has been thoroughly heated. Season and serve at once. Any leftover liquid can add flavor to soups, sauces or gravy.

Eggs

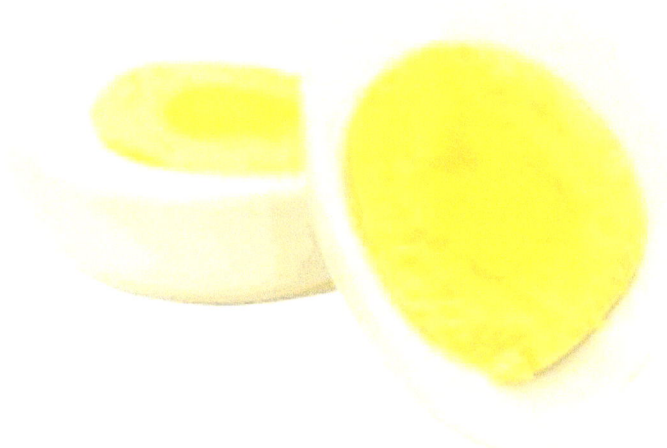

The nutritional value of eggs have been known since ancient times. They are excellent sources of organic proteins, that is why an egg and bacon breakfast was an integral part of the start of the day for centuries in many parts of Europe.

Once upon a time, nobody bothered much about organic eggs because they knew that their eggs supply was coming directly from a farm. But as science and technology began to grow, people started experimenting with eggs, instead of leaving them alone. So now the products you get in the market are eggs, but they have been genetically improved, subjected to scientific procedures and other actions well designed to remove the natural flavor and quality of an egg.

So, if you're lucky enough to find best quality eggs, which are not always available in retail stores, in an organic farm, congratulations! I did not know that eggs were graded into different sizes abroad. In the East, you have just one size, – chicken egg size depending on the poultry variety!

But you are going to find extra-large, large, medium, small and peewee excises in retail stores. These are suitable for frying, soft, hard, and poaching. Some different grades are excellent for cooking and baking.

Cottage Cheese Salad

1 cup cottage cheese, ¼ cup mayonnaise, 2 green onions - chopped, 1 teaspoon parsley, chopped, half a teaspoonful of salt and pepper to taste. I normally add more greens as well as my favorite spices – whichever comes to hand to this salad.

Combine all the ingredients. Serve it on crisp lettuce as an unusual salad or as an item in a fruit or vegetable salad plate.

You can also vary this by substituting canned fruit for the onions and seasonings. Apricots and peaches, as well as pineapple slices are a delicious combination. Combined with mayonnaise and serve.

How to Store Eggs

Whenever possible, by eggs that have been kept under refrigeration. Put them in the refrigerator as soon as possible after you have purchased them. Leave them in the carton with the large end up in a covered container.

Tips on Cooking Eggs

If the eggs are cooked in water, cook under boiling point. If they are baked or fried use low temperatures, high heat will make them tough and unappetizing stop.

Soft Cooked Eggs

Put the eggs in boiling water to cover. Remove saucepan from heat and let stand 5 to 8 minutes. I found the perfect egg recipe from a friend of mine. She used to boil water, and then take it off the heat. And then she used to slip the eggs in it and say the 23rd Psalm. The eggs were done when she finished her prayers. Such an excellent way to get perfectly cooked eggs and getting such a nice start to the day, through prayer.

You can also cover the eggs with cold water and bring to a boil. There is always the danger that the eggshell is going to crack. So put a little bit of salt in the water or even some vinegar. If the eggshell is already cracked, just put some vinegar in the water and you are not going to have spreading egg.

Remove at once for soft cooked or coddled eggs. For medium cooked eggs, remove the pan from the heat and leave eggs in the water for 3 – 5 more minutes.

Hard cooked eggs

Put the eggs in boiling water to cover. Cover saucepan and did you see to keep the waters below simmering for 15 to 20 minutes. Or you can put the eggs in cold water. Cover and heat to boiling. Then set the pan off heat for 20 minutes.

Cool the hard cooked eggs in cold water, as soon as the cooking time is complete. Prompt cooling will prevent overcooking. It will also help prevent the dark ring, which sometimes appears around the Yolk and help the eggshell come off more easily. You can peel the egg easily by starting to peel it at the large end of the egg.

Poached eggs

Fill a shallow pan or frying pan, three quarters full of boiling salted water. Bring the water back to a boil. Break the egg into a saucer, then slip it gently into the water. Repeat with other eggs. A well-drained, attractively poached egg is cooked below the boiling point in salted water. Reduce heat and simmer, covered, for 3 to 5 minutes or until **the eggs are** set to the desired firmness. Lift the eggs out of the water with a slotted spoon or an egg lifter. Drain well and serve on a warm plate on hot buttered toast.

Fried eggs

Fried eggs are delicious when they are fried in the fat which is left over after you have already fried bacon. Slide the eggs gently from a saucer into the hot fat. And yes, the heat to cook the eggs slowly for 3 to 4 minutes. Cover the pan or baste with the fat or turn egg once during cooking, if you are an expert cook to get the pink delicious yolk.

Scrambled eggs

In the frying pan, melt 1 teaspoonful of bacon fat or butter for each egg. Beat the eggs until the whites and the yolks are well mixed. Season with salt and pepper and add 1 teaspoonful of cream, milk, for each egg.

Pour the mixture into the hot fat and cook slowly. Stir gently until the mixture thickens, but is still moist. Serve at once.

Basic French omelets

bacon fat, 5 eggs, 5 teaspoonful cream or milk, half teaspoonful salt and few grains of pepper

Melt the fat in the frying pan, beat the eggs, only enough to mixed white and you ask. Add the seasonings and the liquid. Done. The egg mixture into the frying pan. Reduce heat. As the omelet cooks, prick the bottom and raise the sides to let the liquid portion on the top run underneath until the egg is cooked.

When the bottom of the omelet is lightly browned, fold and turn out on a hot platter. Garnish with parsley. Serve at once. For 4 people.

Cheese

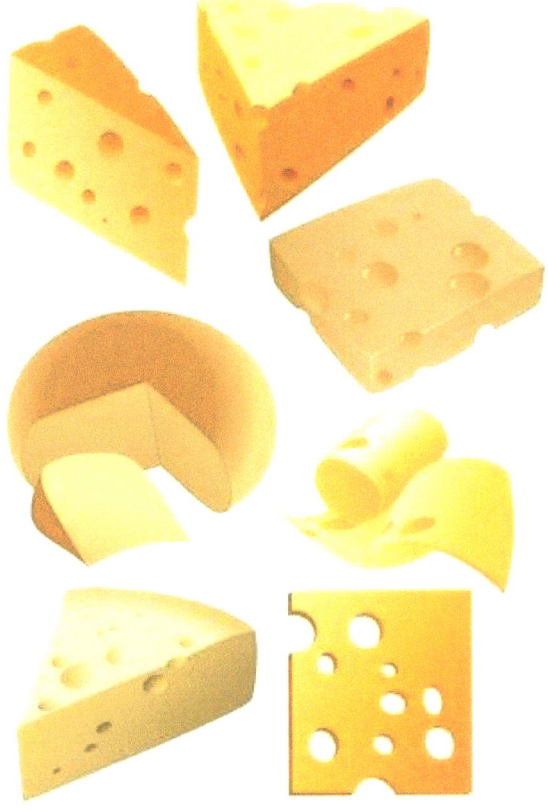

There are many excellent varieties of cheese available in the market today. Some of the most popular of the cheeses available to you in the stores are Parmesan, Swiss cheese, Blue, Gouda and pizza – mozzarella cheese from which to choose.

Cheddar cheese is definitely the most popular of available cheeses, globally, and may be purchased as medium cheddar, mild cheddar, or even old cheddar. The flavor of this cheese is going to vary with the length of time the cheese has been aged. It is delicious and sandwiches, on biscuits, or on a cheese and fruit tray. You can also hire date in sauces and casserole dishes. Half a pound of cheese when grated makes 2 cups

Cheddar cheese is made into many varieties of packaged and processed cheese usually sold under brand names. This processed cheese is smooth textured and maybe grated, sliced or used for spreading. I normally do not advocate eating processed foods, especially when they have chemical preservatives in them. So if you can find a place where somebody makes cheddar cheese at home, or any sort of cheese at home, buy it straight from them. At least he is not going to be putting chemicals in it.

Other hard or semi hard cheeses may be used in the same way as cheddar. These include brick cheese, Swiss cheese, and Gouda

Cottage and cream cheese are the best-known varieties of soft cheese. These cheeses are not aged and are perishable. They may be used for sandwiches, salads, cheesecakes and cheese dips. You may purchase them plain or with a variety of flavorings and seasonings.

 In the East, freshly made cottage cheese is made by professional pastry cooks, to be turned into sweetmeats. It is also made into chunks of 1 pound, which you buy, and take home to add to meat and vegetable dishes.

It is easy to make cottage cheese at home.

https://www.youtube.com/watch?v=at8fSKkRKV4

Noreen has some extremely good videos on her YouTube site, – Noreen's kitchen – where you can also learn butter and yogurt. These are also extremely healthy health foods.

How to Store Cheese

Cook cheese at low temperatures, high temperature is going to toughen cheese.

Cook the cheese sauces over high water to avoid toughening. Add the cheese at the last minute and cook only until it has melted.

Casseroles, which contain eggs, cheese and milk should be poached in the oven in a moderately slow oven. [325 – 3 50°F] . For poaching them in the oven, set the baking dish or the casserole in another pan and surround with hot water.

Cheese and Fruit Tray

You can serve any kind of cheese with crackers, cookies and biscuits. These are attractively arranged on a cheese board, or on a tray or flat serving plate. This is a truly appetizing dessert. Combine different types of cheeses, semi hard and hard, such as cheddar, Swiss and Gouda. Soft cheeses like cream cheese, and processed cheeses and pungent cheeses like blue and Limburger, as well as mild cheeses like Colby and brick cheeses, chopped up in small pieces are good for this fruit tray.

The fruit are going to be slices of apples, fresh pears, cherries, grapes, or any finger fruit available in season. These are a good cheese accompaniment either arranged with the cheese or served separately in a basket or bowl.

You can use this dessert to end a meal or provide the center of attraction at a dessert and coffee party or buffet supper.

Fresh Fruit

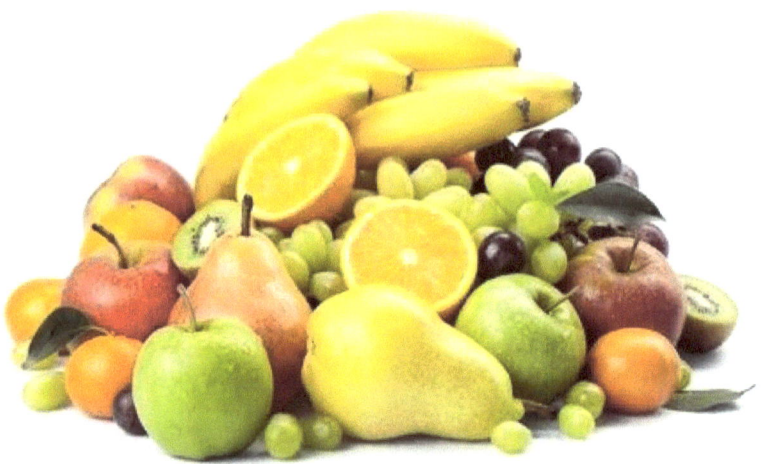

Fruits in one form or the other are available throughout the year and are the simplest and easiest of healthy foods to eat. They are not limited to the dessert course, but can also make attractive, salads, appetizer and between meal snacks. According to the dietitian's food guides, 2 servings of fruit every day need to be eaten, including fruits, which are good sources of vitamins C, like lemons and other citrus fruit.

Fresh Fruit Tips

Buy only the amount of fresh fruit that can be used at once, or stored satisfactorily. Gone are those days when one could walk into the nearest orchard or garden and pick fresh fruit off the trees.

A majority of us now rely on green houses and package fruit available in our departmental store's fruit and vegetable section to give us our necessary healthy quota of fresh fruit.

- If you are buying graded fruit, select the grade suitable for your purpose.

- Keep the under ripe fruit at room temperature until they are ready to serve.

- Store the ripe fruit in a cool place, preferably in the refrigerator, except bananas.

- Wash all the fruit, well before storage and serving. Firm fruits may be washed before storing and soft fruits, especially berries before serving.

- Apples and bananas darken when cut. They should be sprinkled with lemon juice to prevent this exposure to air.

- Most fruits have a better flavor when you remove them from the refrigerator before serving.

Frozen, Canned and Dried Fruits

I am not talking about dry fruit here, which consist of nuts and seeds. Many variety of canned fruits are readily available everywhere and are graded according to their quality. Frozen fruits should be kept continually frozen until just this or use. The best frozen fruits are served while a few ice crystals still remain.

Dried fruits cooked in a shorter time, if you soften them by soaking them in water before cooking. Cook them in the water in which they are soaked.

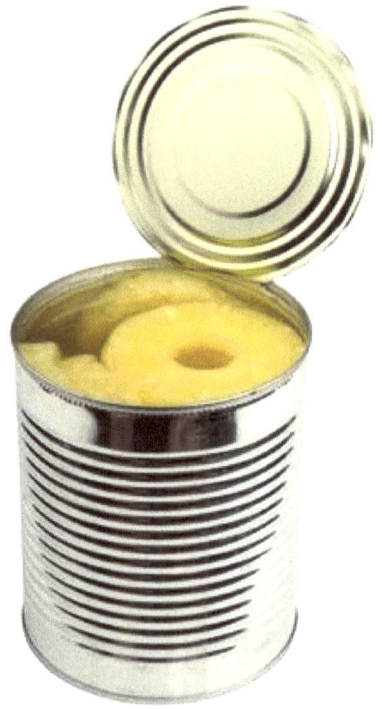

These canned fruit have preservatives. So can and preserve them at home if you can- no pun intended.

Fruit juices are best drunk fresh, but if you are using processed juices, and read the labels to see whether vitamin C has been added to the canned, reconstituted and frozen fruit juice. Pure juices will not need to state their natural vitamin content.

Seriously, I use canned goods only when absolutely necessary, when I have access to fresh fruit. However, canned goods are good as a standby when you could not go to the market or fresh fruit are exorbitantly priced.

Fruit Cup

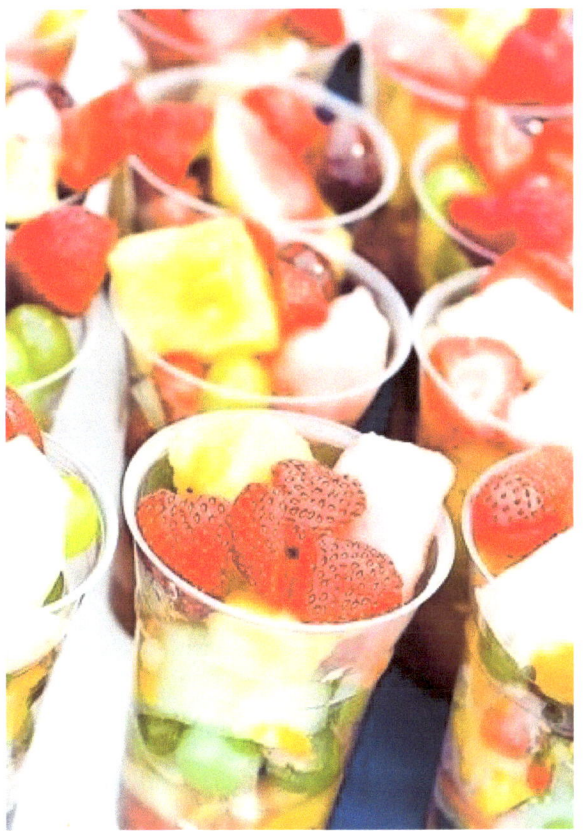

This is a good idea if the fruit is fresh.

Use any attractive combination of fresh fruits to make fruit cups. Chill and prepare for serving. Sweeten if necessary with natural Maple syrup or with powdered sugar. You can also use the sugar used in the canned fruit.

Garnish with nuts, red cherries, old berries or a sprig of fresh mint.

These are excellent combinations –

Sliced fresh peaches, pears and blue berries with a dash of lemon juice

Diced red Apple – unpeeled, sections of grapefruit and peaches

Melon balls or cubes, strawberries and raspberries and sections of orange.

Watermelons

Watermelons are definitely my favorite summer fruit, not only because they prevent dehydration, but they are also good for lowering blood pressure. Be sure to pick up a watermelon when you go shopping, because according to the Florida State University watermelons and cantaloupes can significantly reduce your blood pressure, especially if you are overweight.

The pressure on the aorta and on the heart is going to degrees after you consume watermelons. Watermelon extracts are available in the market today, but bite into a fresh watermelon.

According to this study by the F. S. U. more people died of heart attacks in cold weather because the stress of the cold temperatures caused the blood pressure to increase. The heart then needed to work harder to pump blood to the aorta. This often leads to less than blood flow to the heart.

Eating watermelon, according to this study significantly helps lower the blood pressure and thus prevents potential heart attacks. This study was published in the American Journal of hypertension.

Apples

An Apple a day, definitely keeps the doctor as well as the dentist away. So try these Apple dishes using grandma's traditional recipe.

Baked Apples

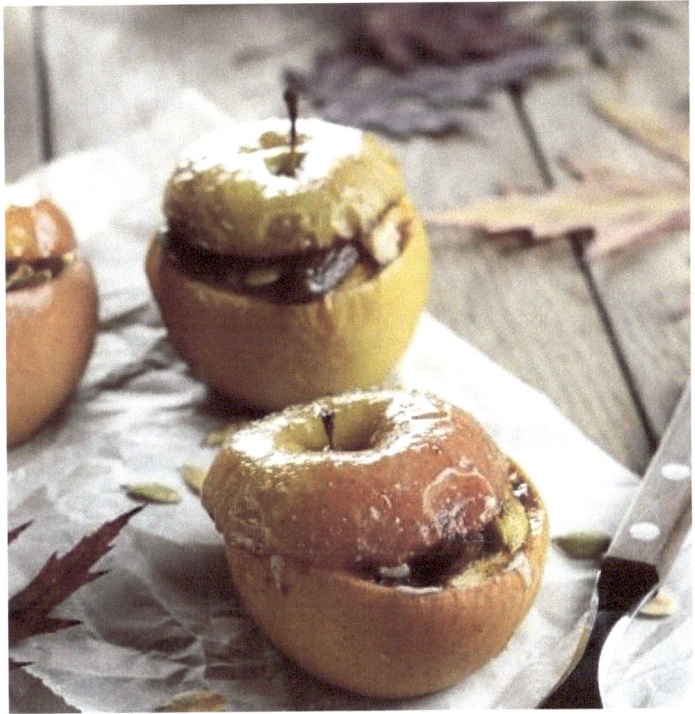

Wash and core large cooking apples. To prevent the skin from breaking, you can score them all a roundabout 1/3 of the way down.

Place them in a shallow baking dish. Fill the center of the apples with ½ – 2 tablespoons full of sugar – Brown for preference. I spiced up the sugar with ¼ teaspoon cinnamon for each ¼ cup sugar. You can also fill the centers with dry fruit mincemeat, raisins or cranberry sauce. Adjust the amount of sugar accordingly.

Top with a little butter and pour enough of water in the dish to prevent in the apples from sticking.

Bake in a moderate oven – 350°F for 35 to 40 minutes or until the apples are tender. Keep basting 2 or 3 times with the liquid in the baking dish. Serve cold or warm with or without cream. When the apples are baked, you can also top each of them with a marshmallow and return briefly to the oven to brown lightly.

Applesauce

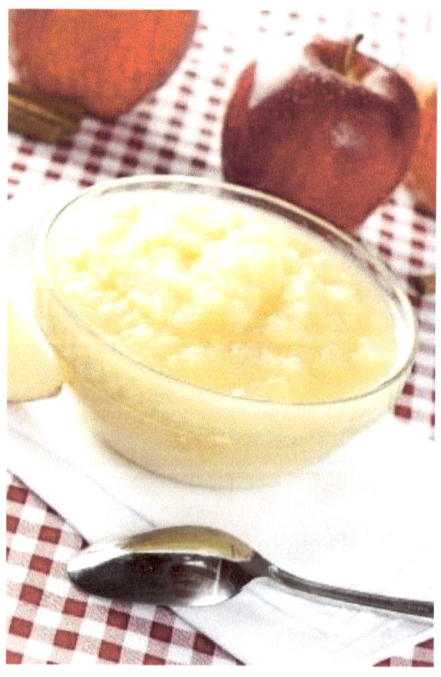

8 cooking apples, 2/3 cup water, ½ cup sugar, 1 teaspoon lemon juice, ¼ teaspoon nutmeg and cinnamon.

Wash water and core the apples. You may leave them unpeeled. Add the water and cook until the apples are soft.

Add sugar, stir until dissolved. When soft, pressed through sieve, sweeten and flavor. Serves 6.

Fish

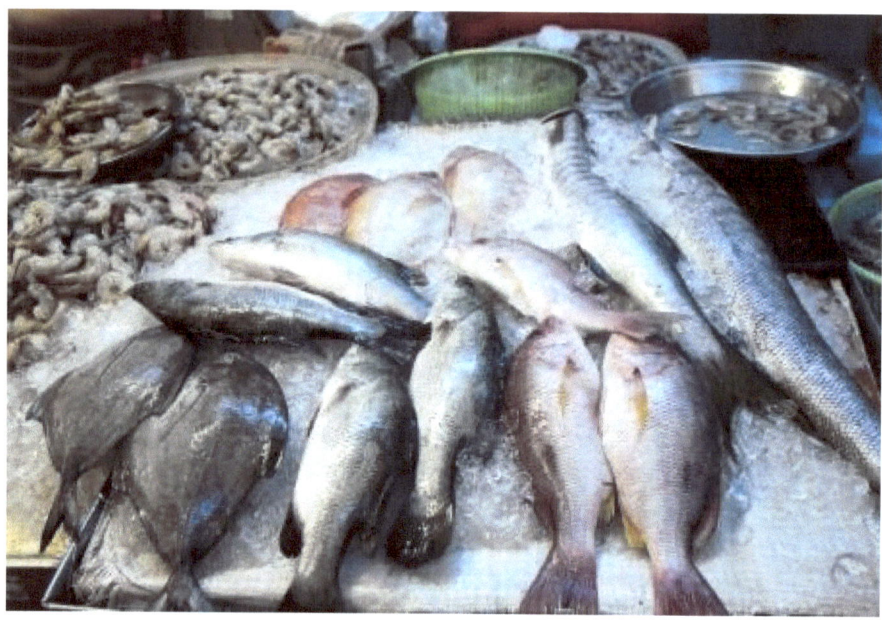

Fish is an extremely good source of omega-3 oil. This is good for your cholesterol and for your heart. Fish is available all throughout the year, fresh or frozen, smoked, dried, and canned. It is a popular alternative to meat and poultry as a main course, organic protein food.

Fresh fish should be cleaned as soon as it has been caught – if you are a keen fisherman – and kept on ice or under refrigeration. It should be used as soon as possible. Frozen fish is hard frozen until ready to cook and when once defrosted, you should not put it back into the freezer.

1 pound per serving is allowed for whole fish. For fish that have been trimmed with the head, tail, and the fins off, allows half a pound per serving. For fish, steaks and fillets allow half a pound per serving.

Cooking Fish the Healthy Way

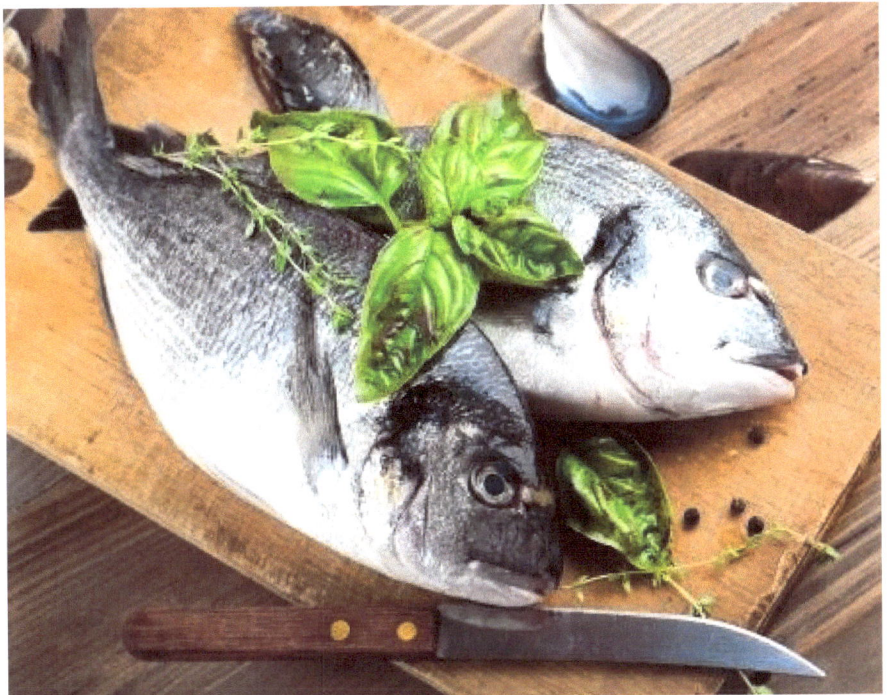

Wash the fresh fish thoroughly in running cold water, drain and pat dry. Frozen fish may be cooked in water or fat without defrosting beforehand. Whole fish which you want to stuff or bake is thawed in its wrappings, overnight in the refrigerator or at room temperature for a shorter time.

Fish unlike meat may be cooked at relatively high temperatures. Steaks and fish fillets may be cooked in an oven at 450°F or pan fried or broiled. You can bake it dipped in salt and milk or plain and coated with fine crumbs or with flour.

Broiling fish can be done by placing it 2 – 4 inches away from the heat. Pan frying is done by a frying it in a frypan with about 1/8 inch of hot fat.

Allow 10 minutes per inch thickness for fresh fish, 20 minutes for frozen fish and small whole fish, fillets and steaks.

Allow 10 minutes per inch thickness for stuffed whole fish and bake at 450°F. Fish is done when the flesh becomes opaque and flakes easily.

Baked Fish Steaks and Fillets

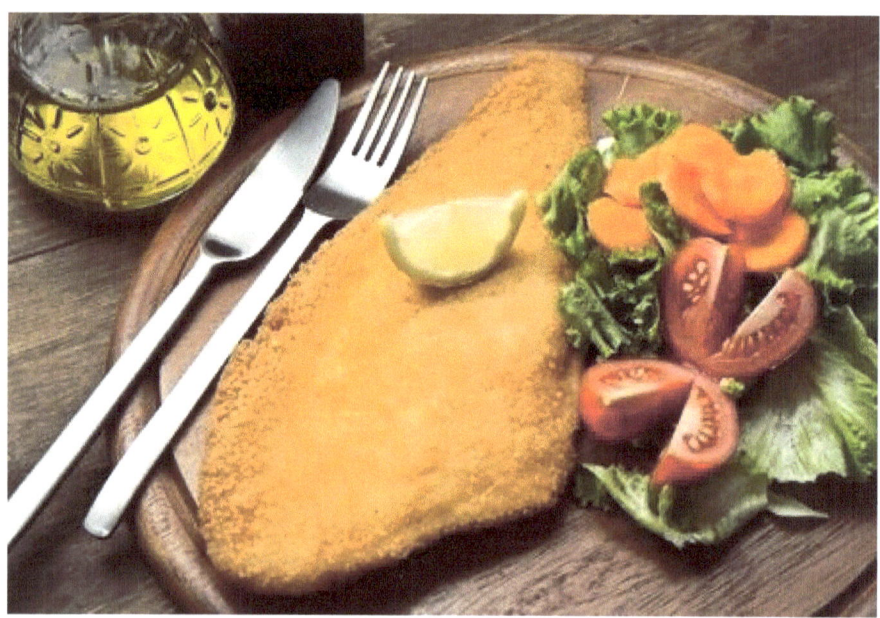

Dip the fish pieces and salted milk – one teaspoonful of salt to ¼ cup milk. Shake off the excess liquid.

Coat with dry bread crumbs or packaged coating mix. Place in a lightly oiled baking pan and sprinkle with a little cooking oil.

Bake in a very hot oven – 450°F for 10 minutes per inch thickness, or until the fish flakes easily with a fork.

Broiled fish

This is extremely good for all those people who are not allowed to eat fried fish due to health reasons. It does not mean that this food items should be boring and bland.

Select small sized whole fishes, fillets and steaks. Sprinkle with salt and if desired, your preferred spices, a few drops of lemon juice and vinegar. I also like to add some garlic to add zing to the broiled mixture. Brush lightly with melted butter.

Place on greased rack under a hot broiler, 2 – 4 inches from the heating unit. Leave the oven door slightly ajar, unless the manufacturer's directions state otherwise. Cook for about 6 minutes, turning fish occasionally and continue cooking until the fish flakes easily with a fork, about 5 to 7 minutes longer. Thin cuts of fish may be broiled without turning.

Frozen fish should be placed 6 – 8 inches away from the heating unit to prevent overcooking the surface before the inside is cooked. Allow a few minutes more cooking time.

Baked Stuffed fish

Wash and dry trimmed fish – 3 pounds will do. Sprinkle the inside and out with salt. Stuff the fish loosely with stuffing. [I am going to give you the stuffing recipe underneath this recipe.] Fasten the cut edges together with skewers or tie with a piece of string.

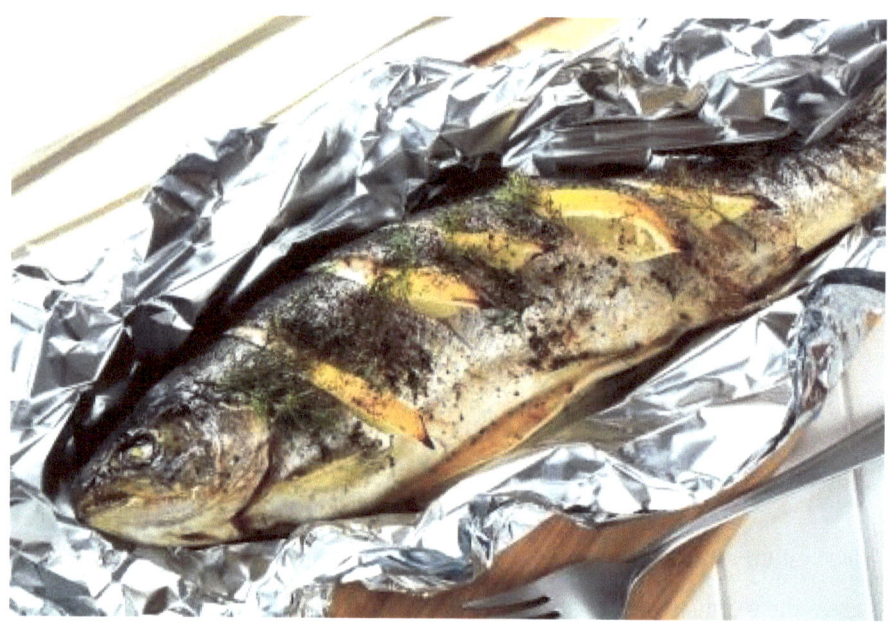

Place the fish in a greased baking pan. Brush with melted oil or butter. I always choose butter, well, because I like it in large quantities like Julia Child! Bake at 450°F. Allow 10 minutes per inch of stuffed thickness until the fish flakes easily. Baste during baking with additional fat if the fish dries out.

Serve with slices of lemon and parsley garnish, and also a sauce if desired.

Bread stuffing

1 ½ tablespoon chopped onion

¼ cup diced celery

3 tablespoon butter

2 cups of soft bread crumbs

Half a teaspoonful of salt with a few grains of pepper

Half a teaspoon each of mixed spices like sage, thyme, basil, Savory and your preferred green or dried herbs.

Cook the onion and the celery in the butter until it is soft.

Add the remaining ingredients and combine. Moisten if you want, with a little bit of milk. Use this stuffing for your fish.

Poached fish

This is a very popular and healthy way either to serve plain or with a sauce or to use for casseroles, salads, or creamed fish dishes. You can also use this for fish cakes.

Measure the thickness of the fish at the thickest part. Sprinkle with salt and lower into boiling water. For ease in removing the cooked fish, place in a wire basket or a wrap of cheesecloth or aluminum foil.

Cover and simmer allowing 10 minutes per inch weakness for fresh fish, and about 20 minutes per inch thickness for frozen fish.

Court Bouillon

Fish either unwrapped or in cheesecloth, may be poached in a seasoned liquid. This is normally called "court bouillon" and is an essential part of French cookery.

Combine a quart of water, half a cup of vinegar, 1 tablespoon full salt, a few celery leaves, 1 sliced onion, a bay leaf, 3 or 4 peppercorns and ¼ teaspoon

Conclusion

These are just some of the healthy basic tips and techniques, which have been passed down the ages to keep you healthy through eating fresh foods cooked properly. Remember most of these tips are common sense. For a proper well-balanced diet, you need to have some food from 5 groups eaten daily. All this should be taken in regular 3 meals a day, even though eating habits are changing with the growing popularity of missed meals, midnight snacks, coffee breaks or dieting.

So do not overlook these food groups, when the day's intake is considered. Good wholesome food will be around for a long time yet, even though most of us are relying on completely little nutritional packages with preservatives and supplements instead of the real thing.

Different kinds of foods have different food values, which mean a varied diet is necessary to provide the necessary proteins, vitamins, minerals and energy. The body requires these essential items to keep functioning properly.

So, make sure that your diet has plenty of meat, fish and poultry, which are protein. One serving a day is enough. Liver should be eaten occasionally because of its exceptionally high vitamins and iron values. Eggs, cheese, and dried beans may be substituted for meat now and then.

It is a good idea to serve eggs at least 3 times a week if not daily.

Vegetables – potatoes, which are available all year around and are relatively inexpensive are extremely worthwhile suppliers of vitamins and minerals, even though there have got a bad press for being full of carbohydrates. To serving a day of other vegetables are recommended. Cooked green or yellow vegetables for their vitamin A, and raw vegetables in salads or for snacks, so that their vitamin content is not lost in cooking.

Fruit – especially recommended our fruits or juices, which are good sources of vitamin C – oranges, apple juice, grapefruit, tomatoes, cantaloupe, and strawberries.

Breads and cereals – This is the least expensive source of energy which includes breakfast cereals and rice. Use whole grain cereals whenever possible.

Milk – whole or skimmed milk, fresh or canned, milk is the food which provides calcium. So make sure that your kids up to 11 years or so get around to and a half cups a day. Teenagers should have 4 cups and adults at least one and a half cups.

Good cooking preserves the natural color of vegetables. It produces the delicate golden brown of nicely fried and baked it gives a rich attractive color to roasted the gravies meets and soups. Poor cooking toughens food, ruins the crisp and tender texture of vegetables, produces lopsided cakes an lumpy sauces, destroys the essential value of food and wastes good food. So the best fun of getting full benefit of healthy meals is cooking it right!

Live Long and Prosper!

Author Bio

Dueep Jyot Singh is a Management and IT Professional who managed to gather Postgraduate qualifications in Management and English and Degrees in Science, French and Education while pursuing different enjoyable career options like being an hospital administrator, IT,SEO and HRD Database Manager/ trainer, movie scriptwriter, theatre artiste and public speaker, lecturer in French, Marketing and Advertising, ex-Editor of Hearts On Fire (now known as Solstice) Books Missouri USA, advice columnist and cartoonist, publisher and Aviation School trainer, ex- moderator on Medico.in, banker, student councilor ,travelogue writer … among other things! One fine morning, she decided that she had enough of killing herself by Degrees and went back to her first love -- writing. It's more enjoyable! She already has 48 published academic and 14 fiction- in- different- genre books under her belt.

When she is not designing websites or making Graphic design illustrations for clients , she is browsing through old bookshops hunting for treasures, of which she has an enviable collection – including R.L. Stevenson, O.Henry, Dornford Yates, Maurice Walsh, C.N.Williamson, Sapper, Bartimeus and the crown of her collection- Dickens "The Old Curiosity Shop," and so on… Just call her "Renaissance Woman" - collecting herbal remedies, acting like Universal Helping Hand/Agony Aunt, or escaping to her dear mountains for a bit of exploring, collecting herbs and plants, and trekking.

Check out some of the other JD-Biz Publishing books

[Health Learning Series](#)

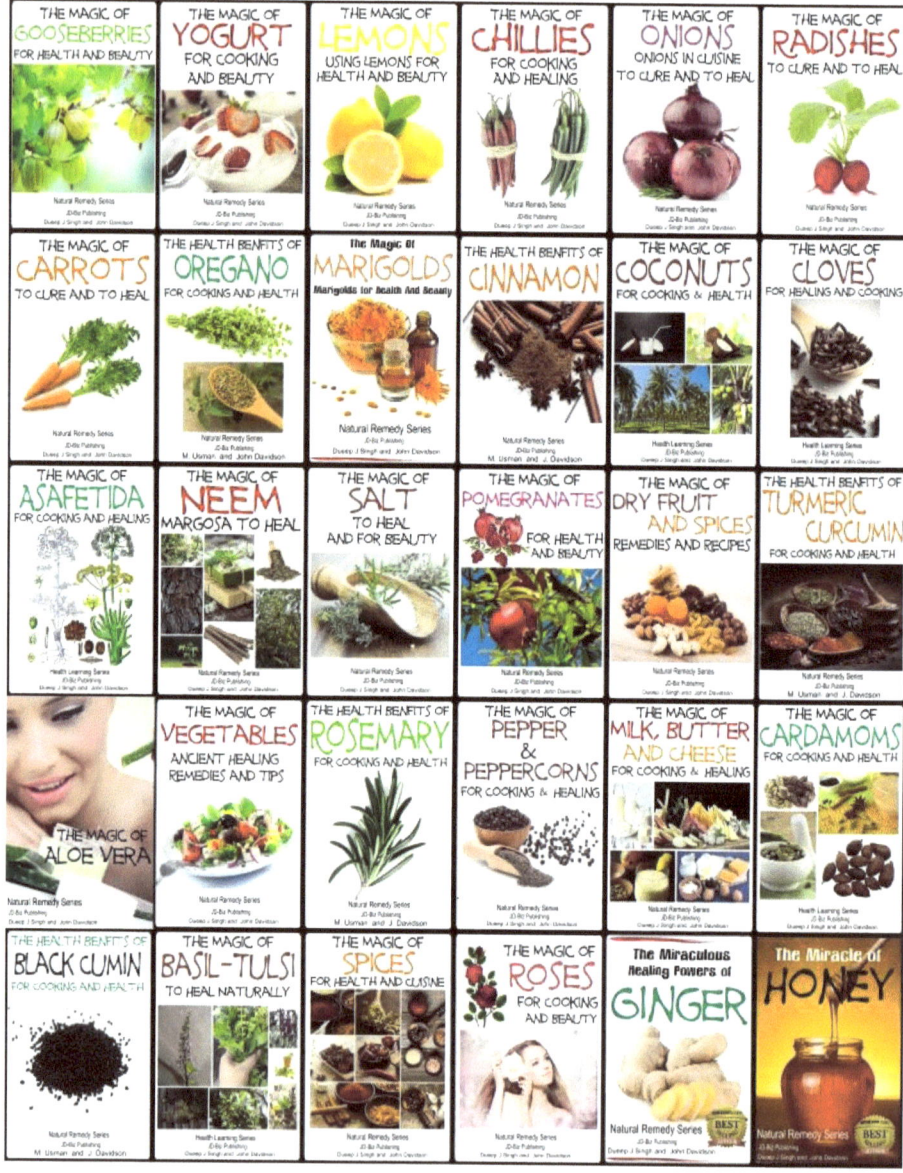

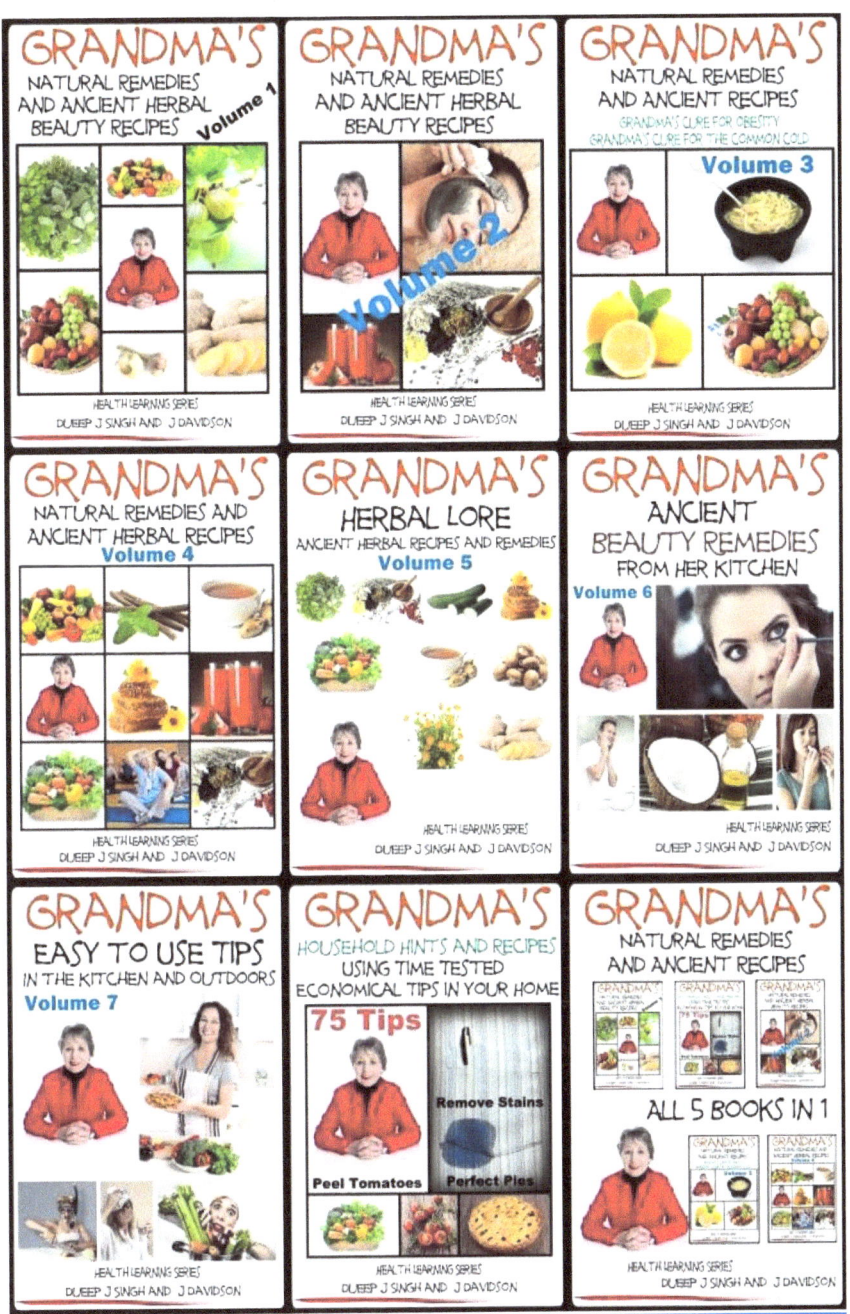

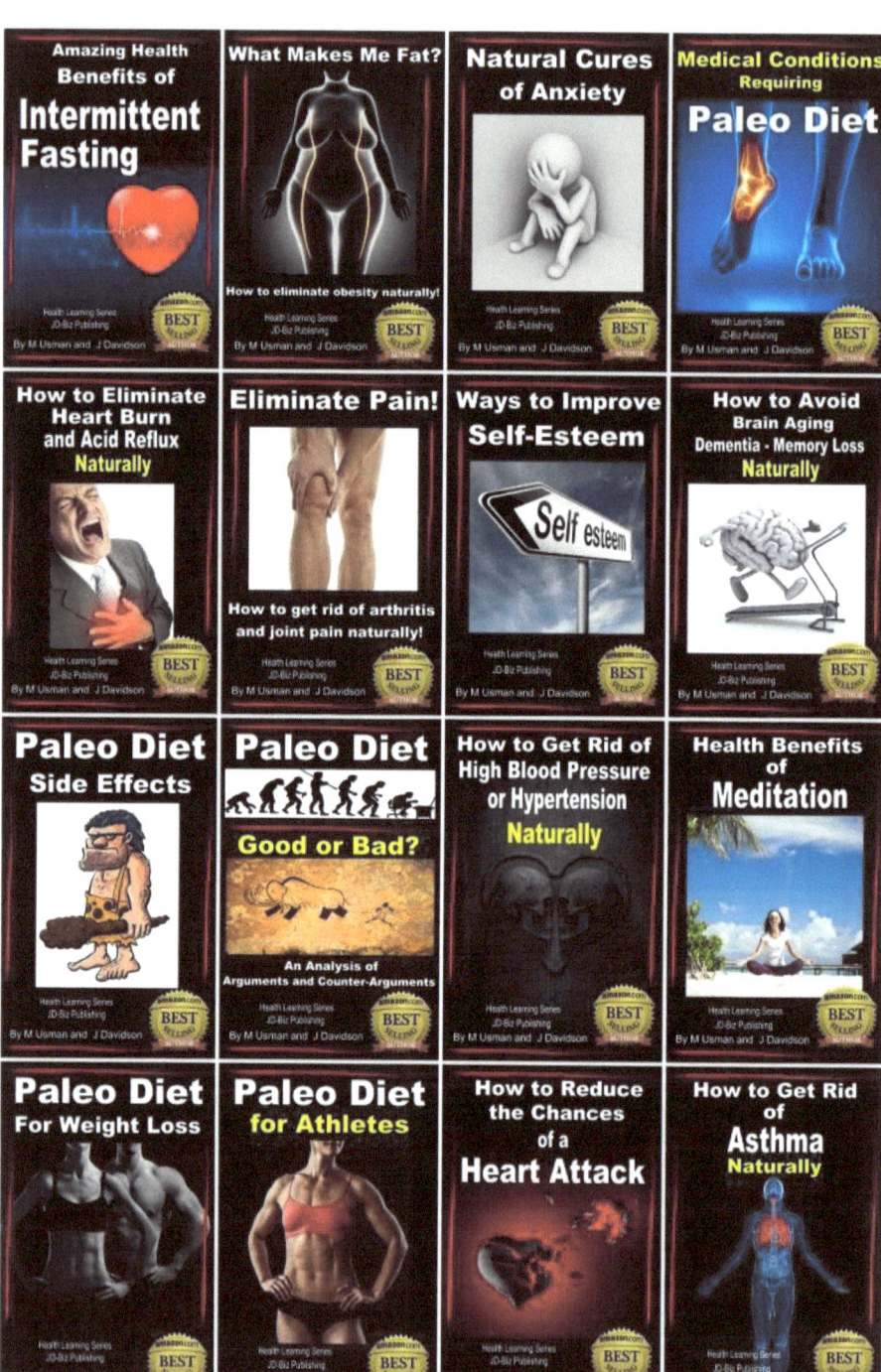

Amazing Animal Book Series

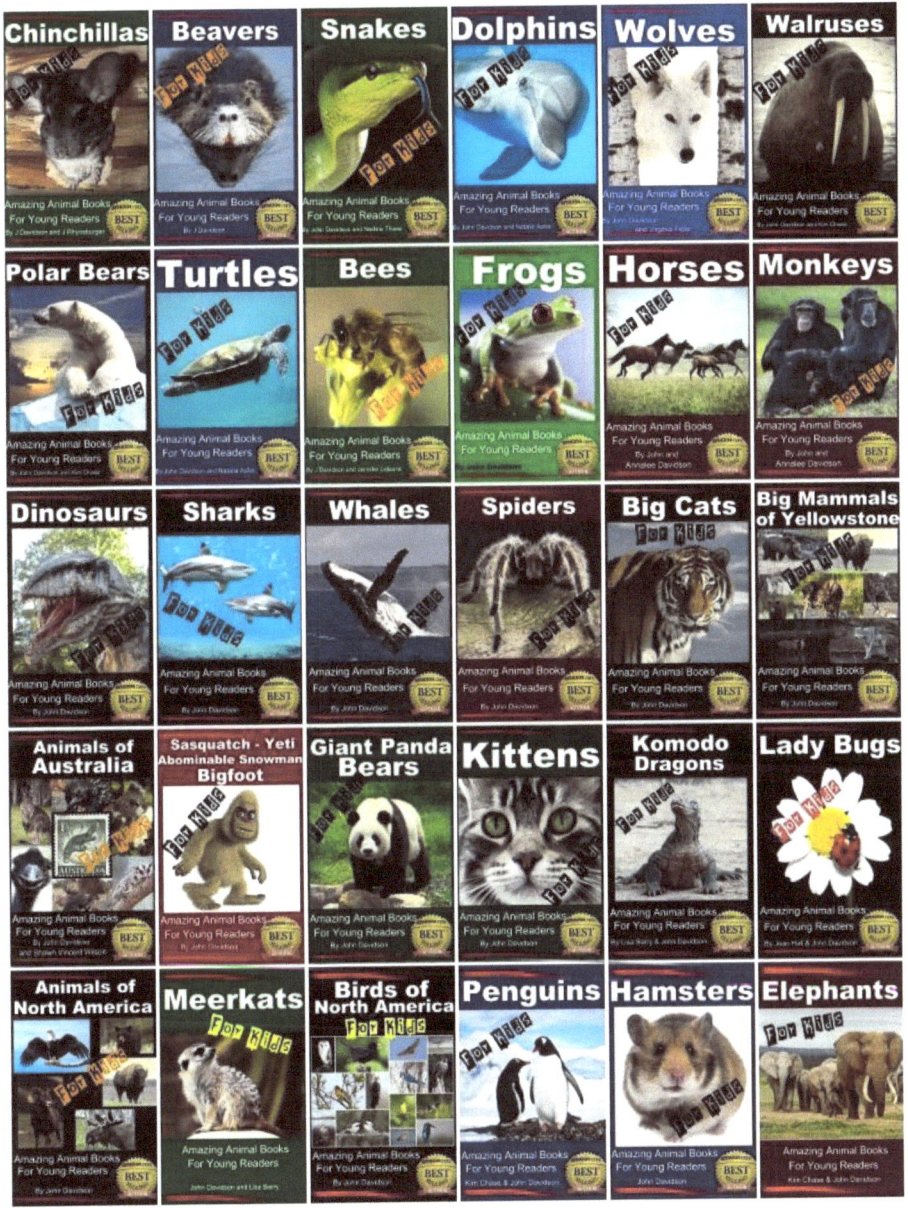

Learn To Draw Series

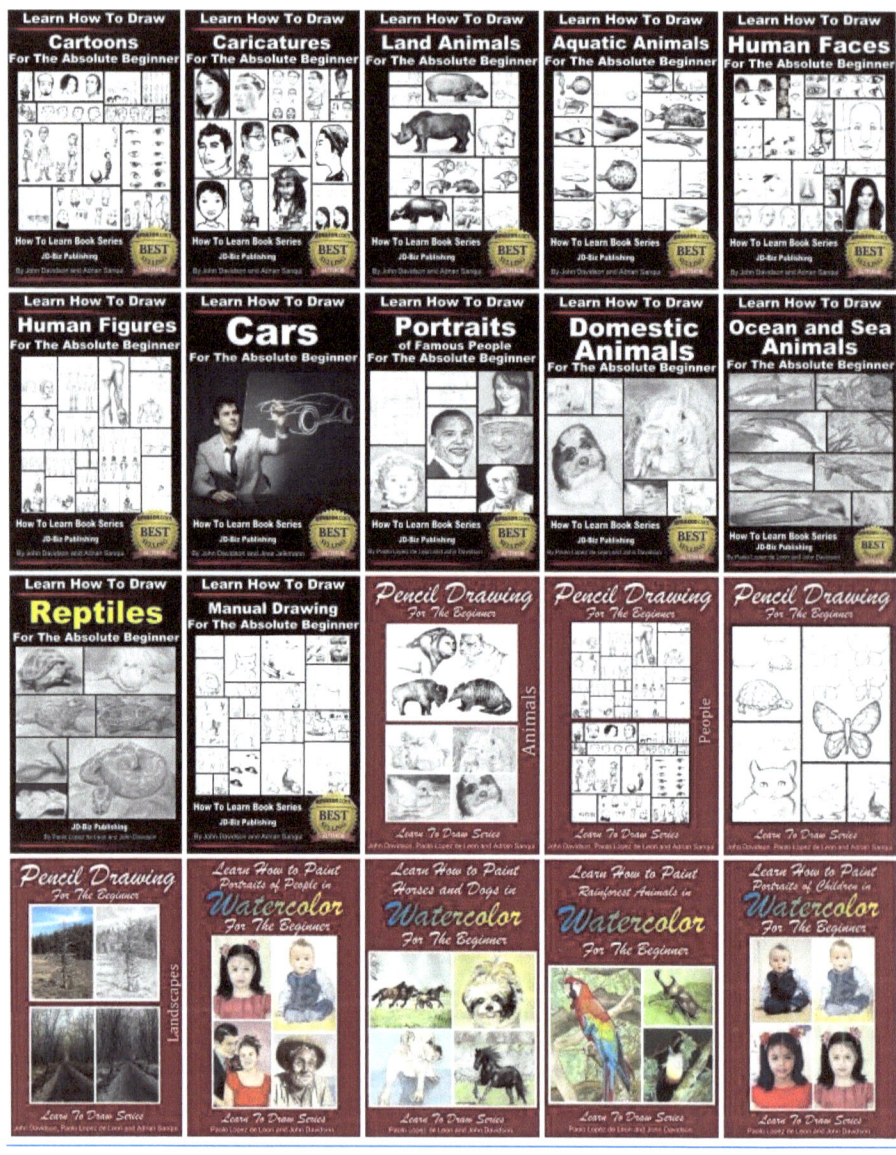

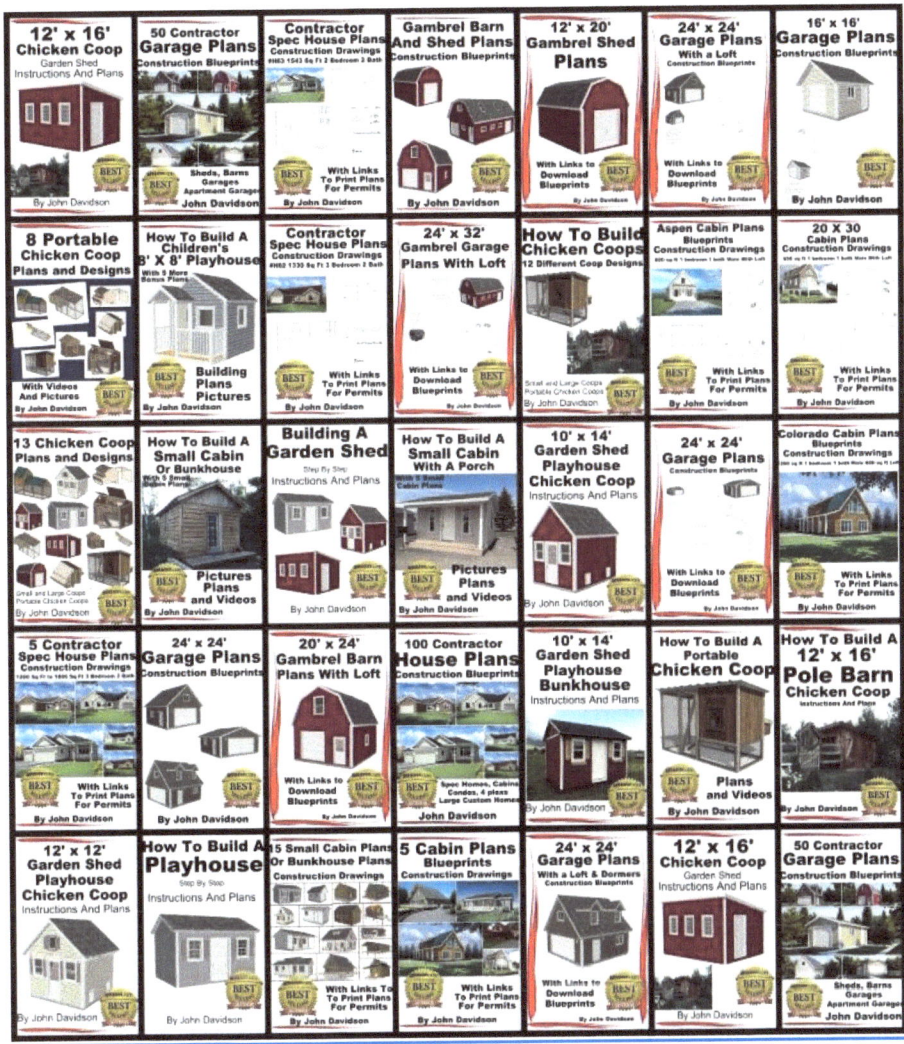

Entrepreneur Book Series

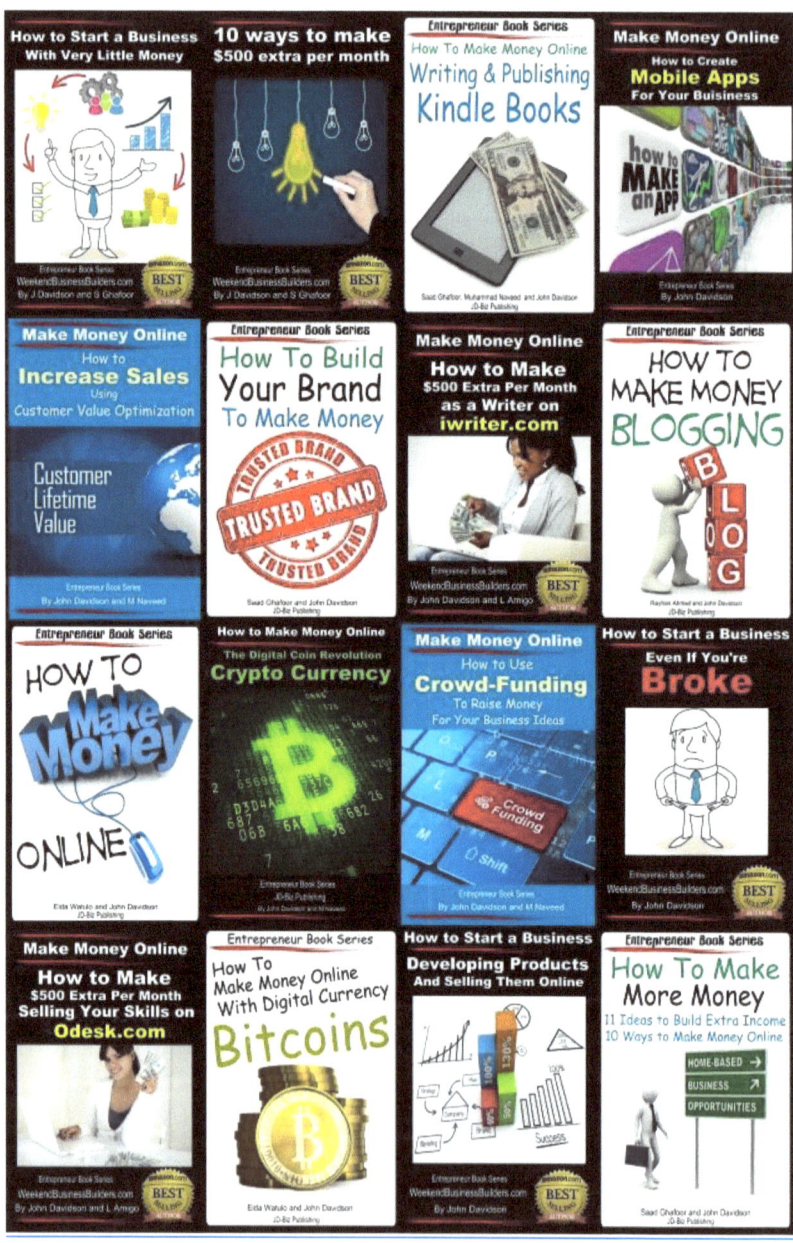

thyme or savory. Cover and boil for 3 minutes before adding fish. Cook as you would do poached fish.

Pan Fried Fish

This is for all those people who love fish and chips. Delightfully greasy, but if you are eating healthy, do not add butter. Small whole fish, fish, steaks, and fillets cut into serving pieces may be pan fried. Partially thaw the frozen fish. Season with salt-and-pepper. Dip in milk or in an egg beaten with 1 tablespoon full of milk. Roll in flour, sifted bread or even cracker crumbs or cornmeal.

Heat shortening in the fry pan. If you are not counting your calories, use bacon fat or butter to cover the bottom of the fry pan well. Do not let the fat smoke.

Add fish. Fry quickly on one side until it is crisp and golden. This will take 2 or 3 minutes. Then turn and cook until the fish flakes easily with a fork but is still moist.

This is how you can get your daily ration of omega-3 rich protein in your diet, and in a healthy manner.

Our books are available at

1. Amazon.com

2. Barnes and Noble

3. Itunes

4. Kobo

5. Smashwords

6. Google Play Books

Download Free Books!

http://MendonCottageBooks.com

Publisher

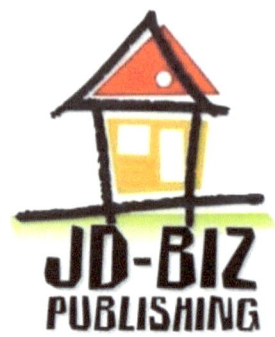

JD-Biz Corp

P O Box 374

Mendon, Utah 84325

http://www.jd-biz.com/

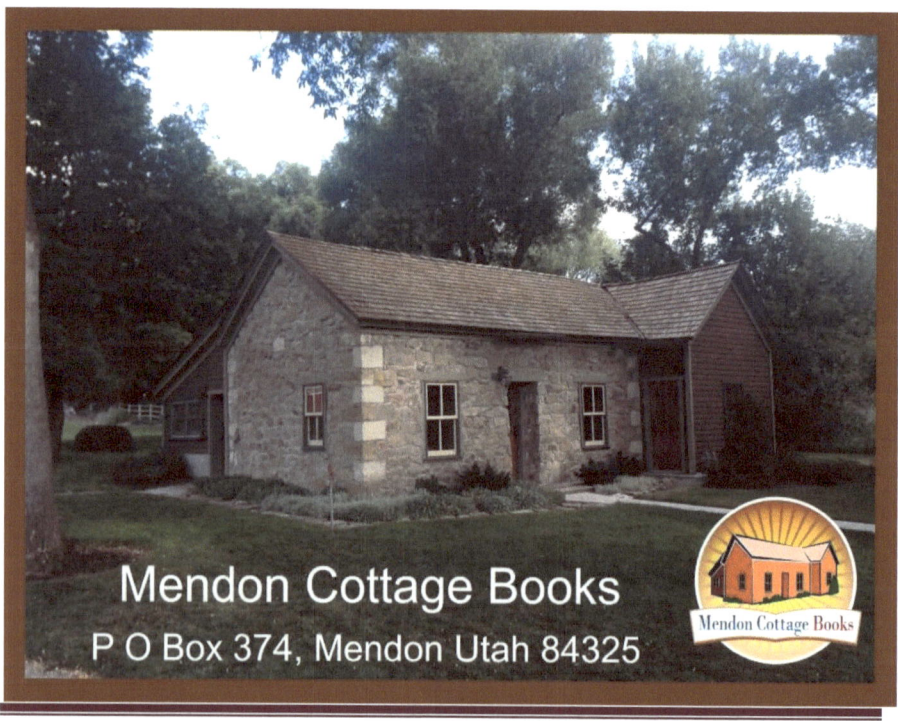

www.ingramcontent.com/pod-product-compliance
Lightning Source LLC
Chambersburg PA
CBHW050828290526
45792CB00001B/308